# DASH Diet

*The Dash diet for beginners, DASH recipes, and teaching you how to lose weight with DASH fast!*

# Table of Contents

Introduction ..................................................................................... 3

Chapter 1: What is the Dash Diet? ............................................ 4

Chapter 2: The Dash Diet Eating Plan ..................................... 10

Chapter 3: Pros and Cons of the DASH Diet ......................... 22

Chapter 4: DASH Diet FAQ ...................................................... 26

Chapter 5: Breakfast Recipes .................................................... 31

Chapter 6: Lunch & Dinner Recipes ....................................... 45

Chapter 7: Smoothie Recipes .................................................... 65

Conclusion .................................................................................... 70

# Introduction

Thank you for taking the time to pick up this book about the DASH diet!

This book covers the topic of the DASH diet (Dietary Approaches to Stop Hypertension) and will teach you all about the diet and its many health benefits!

You will soon learn about why the DASH diet was created, what its many benefits are, the different pros and cons, and also a range of strategies to help you get the best results.

For your convenience, this book also includes some meal planning tips, and a range of different DASH diet recipes to choose from!

At the completion of this book you will have a good understanding of the DASH diet, and will be ready to make the change to a healthier lifestyle!

Once again, thanks for taking the time to read this book. I hope you find it to be helpful, and wish you the best of luck in your new, healthier lifestyle!

# Chapter 1:
# What is the Dash Diet?

Did you know that an estimated 68 million adults in the United States suffer from high blood pressure? This issue is the leading cause of death and also increases the chance of both stroke and heart disease. In the darkness of this issue, there is a light at the end of the tunnel. There are steps you can take to prevent the issue of high blood pressure. We wish to introduce to you, the DASH diet.

DASH diet stands for Dietary Approaches to Stop Hypertension. This diet was developed by the National Heart, Lung, and Blood institute who is based in the United States. Just recently, the DASH diet was named one of the healthiest diets in the United States according to a panel of doctors.

The DASH diet was voted on its effectiveness based upon seven categories. These categories include: ease to follow, nutritional value, safety, short-term weight loss, long-term weight loss, management and prevention of diabetes and the prevention of heart disease. The best part is that this diet was even endorsed by the American Heart Association.

The DASH diet has been scientifically proven to lower blood pressure, lower high cholesterol, and reduces the risk of heart disease. This diet even works to ward off diabetes. As if these weren't already wonderful benefits of being on a diet, the DASH diet offers a strategic way to lose excess weight. This is one of the main reasons why the diet has become so popular. However, it hasn't always been a diet that was designed to be a weight loss program.

While on the diet, people were losing an average of five pounds in their first two weeks. Then over the next two months, an average of 10 to 35 pounds was the reported loss. It should be noted that these results will vary from person to person. It is believed that this weight loss comes from the diet's focus on eating foods that are healthier for us. These foods are lean proteins and healthy fats which give us the feeling of being full. When we are full, this helps us control our appetites so we do not over eat. In the next chapter, we will be going over some more specific details on the foods included in the DASH diet.

## DASH Diet for High Blood Pressure

As you could probably imagine, having high blood pressure is incredibly unhealthy. If your blood pressure is above normal levels, this could increase the chances of having other health risks. Luckily, there are some steps you can take in order to gain control of your high blood pressure. This includes: maintaining a healthy weight, following a healthy eating plan, limiting your alcohol intake, adding physical activity to your daily routine, and taking medication if it has been prescribed by a physician.

If you suffer from high blood pressure, this is where the DASH diet really comes into play. By following the diet's rules, it will help promote a much healthier life. Here are some of the restrictions you will adhere to if you decide to follow the DASH diet:

## Sodium Intake

While on the DASH diet, you will be required to reduce the salt and sodium in your diet. This is due to the fact that salt makes your body retain water. If you take too much sodium into your body, the extra fluid that becomes stored is the reason your body raises your blood pressure. If you take in too much salt while having high blood pressure, it can counteract with blood pressure medicine. On average, adults should not consume more than 6 grams of salt per day. However, many of us consume much more than that limit. The DASH diet will make sure your sodium intake is at a healthy level.

While on the standard DASH diet, the recommended sodium consumption is about 2,300 milligrams of sodium per day. However, if you are on the lower sodium DASH diet, you will only be allowed 1,500 milligrams of sodium per day. Both versions were created to reduce the amount of sodium in your diet. On average, Americans take in about 3,400 milligrams of sodium per day. While the American Heart Association does recommend 1,500 milligrams of sodium per day, this level will vary depending on the person. If you are unsure, you should talk to your doctor and see what your recommended sodium limit should be.

## Fruits and Vegetables

Much like most diets, people lose weight because they are eating healthily. Fruits and vegetables are full of the minerals, vitamins, and fiber that you need in order to keep your body in excellent condition. Some fruits contain potassium which is needed to balance the negative effects that salt has on your body. Through eating these healthy foods, it will have a direct effect on your blood pressure, and will even help lower it after following the diet for a while.

## Magnesium, Potassium, Calcium

On the DASH diet, you will be required to eat foods that are rich in magnesium, potassium, and calcium. Some of these foods include: Skim milk, low fat milk, fat-free and low-fat cheese and even yogurt. These are all major sources of calcium and protein. In the diet plan chapter, you will be learning about all of the foods that will keep you healthy, keep you full, and keep you filled with energy to get you through your day. If you thought all diets were meant to make you miserable, you thought wrong. The DASH diet is all about eating what you want, in healthy proportions. Just because you're on a diet, doesn't mean you need to starve!

## Alcohol

While some of you may be groaning at this point, there is a reason that everything needs to be limited to moderation. If you drink less alcohol, it will help you to avoid high blood pressure. Also, if you weren't already aware, alcohol contains a lot of calories. An excess of calories makes you gain weight. The DASH diet recommends a limit of 21 units of alcohol for men per week and 14 units for women per week. However, if it gives you high blood pressure and makes you gain weight, why bother? There are other healthy alternatives to keep you in tip top shape!

## Fats and Cholesterol

If you have high blood pressure, it is a good idea to cut back on foods that are high in cholesterol and bad fats. By having a low-fat diet, this can help keep you at a healthy weight. If you eat foods that are low in saturated and trans-fats, it also helps keep your cholesterol level down in your blood. When you have too much cholesterol, this is what can increase your risk of getting heart disease or having a stroke. Check out the salt, the sugar, and the saturated fat levels before you buy your food. These are all small steps you can take in order to lower your blood pressure.

## Starting the DASH Diet

The DASH diet normally consists of around 2,000 calories per day. If you are trying to lose weight on this diet, you may need to adjust the number of calories you take in, as every person's caloric needs are different. Remember that the DASH diet wasn't originally created to help people lose weight, but rather to lower blood pressure.

There are some simple strategies to help you get started on the DASH diet. Many people struggle with diets at first, but don't worry, this is totally normal. What we can tell you is that you will not regret starting!

First, you will want to start making the changes gradually. At this point in your life, you probably only eat a couple of servings of fruits and vegetables a day. Instead, try adding a serving of a fruit or a vegetable at lunch time and then another at dinner. Also, if you're stuck on white bread, try to switch to whole grain for one of your meals. By slowly increasing these healthier foods, it can help prevent any bloating and diarrhea that often comes with a sudden change in diet.

If this doesn't work, there are over-the-counter products that will help reduce gas from additional fiber in the vegetables.

Another way to increase weight loss on the DASH diet is to add a physical activity to your daily routine. This can also help boost your efforts in lowering your blood pressure. Try something easy like going for a walk, meditating, or going for a swim at your local pool! You don't have to work hard, just make a simple start and then work your way up to more strenuous activities!

Being on a diet can be very difficult. It is very important that you remember to reward yourself for your success. However, a reward does not always need to be with food. Instead, watch a movie you've been dying to see, or get that new book you've been eyeing. Just remember that everyone slips. This is especially true for those who are trying something new. A diet change is going to be a lifestyle change. You're not just going to suddenly change your habits and become healthy! It is a process. Forgive yourself and pick up where you left off. It's a long journey, but it will be worth it.

Now, for the comprehensive food plan to help you on your way!

# Chapter 2:
# The Dash Diet Eating Plan

If you do happen to suffer from high blood pressure, your doctor may have recommended the DASH diet for you. As we now understand, DASH diet stands for Dietary Approaches to Stop Hypertension. Luckily for you, the diet is incredibly simple. This is probably why the diet has been voted one of the best not only for weight loss, but also for its numerous health benefits.

While on the diet, you will be eating more fruits, vegetables and low-fat dairy foods. As you do this, you will also cut back on the foods that are high in trans-fat, cholesterol, and saturated fat. This can be easy to do because most foods are labeled. You will also want to eat healthy foods such as poultry, fish, whole-grain foods, and nuts. There is a way to diet and still make it delicious. You will just want to make sure that you limit the amount of sweets, red meats, sodium, and sugary drinks you take in. When followed correctly, many people have reported a lowered blood pressure reading within two weeks!

## Starting the Diet

Much like any diet you will find yourself on, the diet will call for a certain number of daily servings from the various food groups. This number will change depending upon how many calories you need per day.

One of the most important aspects to understand is that you will not just be jumping directly into the diet. It has taken years to form your eating habits. By making gradual changes, it won't put your system into shock. For example, try limiting yourself to about 2,400 milligrams of sodium per day. Once your body has adjusted to this limit, go ahead and cut back to 1,500 milligrams of sodium per day. This may sound like a lot, but it is actually only 2/3 of a teaspoon!

While we will be teaching you about what to eat, it is important to understand what a serving is. When you are attempting to follow a healthy eating plan, you must understand that there is such thing as too much of a good thing. Here is a short comprehensive list to follow when choosing your food for the DASH diet.

## One Serving:

| Cooked Rice or Pasta | ½ Cup |
|---|---|
| Raw Fruits and Vegetables | 1 Cup |
| Cooked Fruits and Vegetables | ½ Cup |
| Cooked Meat | 3 Ounces |
| Tofu | 3 Ounces |
| Sliced Bread | 1 Slice |
| Milk | 8 Ounces |
| Olive Oil | 1 Teaspoon |

# Diet Tips

Starting a diet can be very difficult. Whether you are doing this to lower your blood pressure or just to lose weight, know that we are here to help guide you along your path. Remember that it is perfectly fine to slip up every once in a while, just as long as you don't return to your old habits for good. Here are some diet tips to help you along the way. After, we will be giving you an easy food plan to follow to get you started.

1. If you aren't used to having fruits and vegetables as a part of your diet, slowly begin adding them in. We suggest starting out with an extra serving during either lunch or dinner. If this doesn't work for you, you can also add them as a snack between meals. When using canned or dried fruits however, make sure that there is no added sugar!

2. You will always want to read labels when shopping for your food. Of course, the golden rule is to always shop on the outside edges of the grocery store. You will want to shop fresh whenever possible. However, if you do choose food from a can, make sure you choose products that are lower in sodium.

3. Most of us enjoy snacking. Instead of reaching for chips or those incredibly tempting sweets, try to grab something healthier for you. Try low-fat yogurt, frozen yogurt, plain popcorn, raw vegetables, nuts, or even unsalted pretzels. They will keep you full and give you the satisfying crunch you are looking for.

4. If you are a meat eater, try to limit your intake to about 6 ounces per day. If you can, try to make most of your meals vegetarian. This way, you will be eating more healthily and will likely increase the amount of fruits and vegetables you are consuming to compensate.

5. When you can, try to drink skim or low-fat dairy products. This can be a simple switch if you are used to only using full-fat milk or even cream. You can do this by stocking your home with only low-fat and skim products.

6. Portions are a very difficult concept for many people to grasp. When you are first eating on the DASH diet, try to use only half of your typical serving. This stands especially true for condiments and other extras such as margarine, butter, and even salad dressing. Much like the dairy products, reach for low-fat or fat-free when you can to help cut back on extra calories.

## DASH Diet Phases

The DASH diet works in two different phases. The first phase is meant to reset your metabolism and then the second will help to manage your weight loss. It is important to follow the plan as recommended. Remember that this diet is recommended for those who are suffering from hypertension (high blood pressure.) However, this diet also works for those who are trying to prevent kidney stones, certain types of cancer, heart disease, and diabetes. Follow the simple two step plan to reap the many benefits of this diet.

## Phase One

The first phase takes place over 14 days. During this phase, you will be learning all about how to satisfy your hunger. Many people worry that when they're on a diet, they are going to be starved. This is not the case with the DASH diet! By eating the correct foods, it will help regulate your blood sugar and in return, curb your cravings! During this phase, you will want to avoid fruit and whole grains due to the fact that they have a large amount of natural sugars. Also during this phase, you will be avoiding alcohol.

When you are able to avoid all of these starchy foods that are high in sugar, your body will be able to regulate your blood sugar. Instead, reach for leafy greens such as lettuce, spinach, broccoli or cabbage. It is also a good idea to eat foods such as squash, peppers, tomatoes, and even cucumbers. On top of that, you will be able to enjoy lean meats, fish, and even poultry. We suggest anywhere up to 6 ounces per day.

During the first phase, try your best to go for protein-rich foods. Often times, these also come with the benefits of having healthy fats. Try to incorporate fresh nuts and seeds into your diet. Another excellent choice are avocados! These are filled with monounsaturated fats, vitamin E and even beta-carotene. You will find that there are so many different ways to make your diet delicious, you'll wonder why you didn't start sooner!

## Phase Two

In the second phase, you will continue eating the same foods as phase one, but then you will be introducing some other healthy foods. By adding a larger variety of foods, it will help to continue your weight loss. During this phase, your diet choices need to become a lifestyle rather than a diet. As long as you keep up the diet, you will be able to keep your blood pressure low and keep the excess weight off. In this phase, we will introduce healthy whole grains, starchy vegetables, and fruits back into your diet.

Below, we will include some guidelines for keeping your diet in check.

## Daily DASH Diet: Approximately 2,000 calories per day

### Grains – 6 to 8 Servings

Remember that it all comes down to portion size. You can eat healthy foods all day long, but it won't do much for your waist line if you over-eat. Instead, try to eat healthy but in moderation. When we say grains, this includes foods such as bread, cereal, rice, and pasta. Remember that one slice of whole-wheat bread counts as a serving. As for the pasta, rice, and cereal, a serving is about ½ cup. If it is dry cereal, a serving will be 1 ounce.

### Fruits – 4 to 5 Servings

You probably assumed that all fruits are healthy for you. Just remember that some fruits are higher in sugar than others. Most fruits are rich in potassium, magnesium, and fiber. They also have the vitamins and minerals our body needs to function. A serving a fruit is about ½ cup if it is fresh or frozen. If it is a whole fruit, 1 medium sized fruit will be counted as a single serving.

## Vegetables – 4 to 5 Servings

One of the best aspects of vegetables is that they are rich in vitamins and also include the fiber we need in our diet. Vegetables can be delicious and keep you full at the same time. This is why we recommend incorporating as many different fruits and vegetables as you can into the DASH diet. Reach for vegetables such as: sweet potatoes, green beans, tomatoes, carrots, and broccoli. One serving is ½ of a cup if it is raw or cooked and 1 cup for the leafy green vegetables. You will be surprised at how much food this actually is!

## Lean Meat, Poultry, and Fish - 6 Servings

While these foods are rich in proteins, zinc, and B vitamins, we suggest keeping these foods to a minimum. Try to keep most of your diet to fruits and vegetables but use meats, poultry, and fish for a dish every once in a while. One serving of poultry is 1 ounce. This stands the same for seafood and lean meat. If you enjoy eggs, 1 egg is a serving and 1 ounce of tuna from a can is also a serving.

## Dairy – 2 to 3 Servings

As we mentioned earlier, be sure to always keep your dairy either skim or low fat. This is important for your diet because dairy is going to be a major source for protein, calcium, and even vitamin D. Go for foods such as yogurt, milk, and even cheese! One cup of skim milk is equal to one serving. If you want to incorporate yogurt, that is also one cup. As for the cheese-lovers out there, one serving of cheese is equal to 1.5 ounces.

## Legumes, Nuts, and Seeds – 4 to 5 Servings

You may have been told that nuts are bad for you because they are high in calories. However, they are amazing for the essential nutrients our bodies need. From protein, to potassium, fiber, and even magnesium. Try to reach for peas, lentils, almonds, pistachios, peanuts and delicious sunflower seeds next time you need something to snack on. They are even delicious to decorate your salad with!

## Fats and Oils – 2 to 3 Servings

While it may seem strange that you have to incorporate fats and oils into the diet, it should be noted that our body actually needs this fat in order to properly absorb all of the nutrients and vitamins the healthy foods will be giving us. Fats are also great for our immune system. However, only in moderation, and only the correct types of fat. For mayonnaise, one serving is 1 tablespoon. If you are a dressing type of person, 2 tablespoons equals one serving. Always be sure to check out the labels so you don't overdo anything!

## Sweets - 5 Servings PER WEEK

Yes, you read that correctly! There is no reason you need to give up sweets altogether! Sure, if you cut back on sweets, it will help you to lose weight quicker, but sometimes they are just nice to have. Remember that everything is OK in moderation. Try having ½ cup of sorbet, 1 tablespoon of jam/jelly, or even 1 cup of lemonade to cure that sweet tooth.

As you can see, there really isn't much of a difference between your normal eating habits, and the DASH diet. Basically, the eating style just puts emphasis on healthy foods such as fruits, vegetables, and whole grains. Most likely, these are foods that you eat already to some degree! The whole point is to just eat these healthy foods as often as possible, while lowering the quantities of unhealthy ones. Go ahead and try to start with just changing one meal and then you can add another. Success is all about the changes that are made over time. It will require a lot of motivation and some patience.

Here are just a few sample meal suggestions to get you started on your way.

## Breakfast

The way most of us like to start our day before we head to work, school, or anything else. It is said that breakfast is the most important meal of the day. Here are just some ideas to keep it healthy and within the DASH diet guidelines.

1. Our morning coffee. It is the ultimate wake-up solution. Instead of reaching for the cream, try your latte with some fat-free or even low fat milk instead!

2. If you enjoy toast in the morning, reach for some nut butter and then top it with slices of apple, banana, raisins or even pears. This way, you have your bread but also incorporate a serving of fruit in there!

3. Are you more of an omelet person? This is the perfect time to get a serving or two of vegetables into your diet. Add in some chopped onions, spinach,

tomatoes, or even mushrooms to produce a delicious and filling meal.

4. Another excellent breakfast alternative is yogurt! Looking for something a bit more delicious? Make a breakfast parfait. Layer a low-fat yogurt with fresh fruit, granola, and even whole-grain cereal. It will look pretty, and taste delicious!

5. If you're in a hurry, whole-grain cereal can be a good choice. If you have the extra time, try to add slices of banana, fresh berries, or even dried fruit on top.

# Lunch

1. If you normally have a sandwich for lunch, this is perfect. Go ahead and load it up with tomatoes, peppers, carrots, and other delicious vegetables. If you have a deli meat on there, just make sure it is within your serving size.

2. During lunch, it can be tempting to reach for soft drinks or soda to give you the afternoon pep you need to get through the rest of the day. Don't do it! Instead, try drinking skim or low-fat milk to quench your thirst.

3. If you go out for lunch, try to head for the salad bar. There are so many excellent and fresh choices for you to pick from. Most salad bars will also offer soup. Go for the broth-based vegetable or the bean soup if possible.

## Dinner

1. If you are looking for a new way to prepare dinner, try grilling your vegetables! We suggest doing this with mushrooms, eggplant, cauliflower, and even peppers! All you'll need to do is drizzle them with some balsamic vinegar and you are all set to go!

2. When you can, try a vegetarian recipe. Yes, meat can be good every once in a while, but the DASH diet is more about healthier options. There are many delicious recipes out there that won't make you miss red meat.

3. One-pot meals are an excellent way to prepare dinner. Throw in some vegetables, brown rice, some quinoa, and some beans and you are all set. Allow it all to cook in a slow-cooker for the day and you'll have a delicious meal come dinner-time!

4. A stir-fry is another great alternative for those who are looking for more ways to get vegetables into their diet. You can even include small portions of shrimp, tofu or chicken to spice up the recipe.

## Dessert

1. As you may have guessed, fruit is the best option. It will give you something sweet to satisfy those cravings and also keep you full! Be sure to check the natural sugar content of the fruit. Yes, it is healthy but it can also put you over your daily allowance.

2. Fruit kebabs can be a fun way to have dessert, especially if you are trying the DASH diet while having a family. We suggest using chunks of melon, pineapple, and other fruits like grapes and berries to make them colorful and delicious.

The point is, you can have dessert. Just make it healthy!

# Chapter 3:
# Pros and Cons of the DASH Diet

When you follow the DASH diet, this will naturally reduce the consumption of salt you take in. The dietary requirements will vary between people depending on a variety of factors. These include your age, any current and past health conditions you may have. It is also important to be active while on this diet. By being physically active, you will achieve your optimal weight that is healthy for you quicker. If you are overweight, it will further your risk of heart disease and high blood pressure.

Here are some of the key benefits of the DASH diet:

## Weight Loss

This weight loss will be caused by the deficit of calories that come along with the DASH diet. While the diet does not stress calorie reduction, the food plan is filled with nutrient-dense foods that help to shed off any excess weight. Also, the diet is rich in fiber which studies show contributes to weight loss. The key is to optimize your health through nutrients. Even if you do not have a blood pressure issue, the DASH diet is worth incorporating into your daily life.

## Lowered Cholesterol

As you add the additional fiber into your diet with whole grains, this will help to reduce your cholesterol levels. It is suggested that men aim for 38 grams of fiber while women should take in 25 grams per day. While the cholesterol falls, the blood pressure will be reduced as well.

## Reduced Blood Pressure

Through this whole book, you've been reading all about the DASH diet and how it can reduce blood pressure. Just remember that this is largely due to the composition of calcium, potassium, and magnesium. Each of these play a key role in lowering your blood pressure. This is why the DASH diet is filled with so many healthy fruits and vegetables that contain these nutrients. It is however, most important to lower your sodium intake! When there is too much fluid built up, it can cause critical bodily functions. When this additional fluid puts strain on your heart, this increases your blood pressure. Keep it down with the DASH diet!

## DASH Diet Pros

1. DASH foods are very filling. This will help make losing weight so much easier when you are not worried about being hungry all of the time.

2. We encourage enjoyable exercise! You shouldn't hate everything you are doing just to lose weight. As long as you're moving, you're improving!

3. This diet is very heart-healthy. By participating in the DASH diet, you will lower your blood pressure and lower your risk for heart disease.

4. This diet is diabetes friendly! It has been known to lessen the conditions that come with diabetes and can also be used to prevent diabetes in the first place!

5. The DASH diet also does not include any special foods or expensive supplements. The diet is filled with foods you probably already eat and can access easily at your local grocery store!

6. There is a lot of scientific research behind the DASH diet to support the effectiveness. This is why the diet has been rated one of the top of its kind!

7. The DASH diet was even endorsed by places including the American Heart Association, the 2010 Dietary Guidelines for Americans, the Mayo Clinic, and even the National Heart, Lung, and Blood Institute.

8. A great added benefit of the DASH diet is that it has long-term potential. Too many times people do FAD diets for a quick and easy change. The issue is that the results are only temporary. With the DASH diet, it is easy to follow and can be a lifelong change.

## Cons

1. One of the downfalls of this diet is the fact that you need to keep track of what you eat. Remember that portion and serving size is incredibly important. Luckily, there are phone apps to keep this as simple as possible.

2. Some people find that foods that have less salt are pretty flavorless. This is why we suggest sticking with fresh fruits and vegetables, they come naturally delicious! You can also try adding fresh herbs and spices to make your food a bit tastier!

3. The DASH diet requires a lot of fiber. Some people have issues adjusting to taking in so much. We believe it is a good idea to gradually add more fiber to your diet. This way, you can avoid any discomfort or bloating that may occur as a side effect.

# Chapter 4:
# DASH Diet FAQ

## Q: Is the DASH Diet Expensive?

**A:** The answer to this question will vary depending on the area in which you live. The broad answer is that it will generally be more expensive than eating junk. This is because any fresh fruits, vegetables, and whole grain products are normally a bit pricier than processed foods. We believe that for your health, it will be worth it!

## Q: Will I really lose weight on the DASH Diet?

**A:** As explained earlier, this diet wasn't really developed as a weight-loss diet. However, studies have shown that DASH does have the potential to help shed excess weight. One example was published in the Archives of Internal Medicine in 2010. The studies were on 144 overweight adults who had high blood pressure. These individuals were assigned to either DASH, DASH plus exercise, or just be on a controlled diet with the usual eating habits. After four months, the DASH groups with exercise lost an average of 19 pounds. The other two groups lost a little bit of weight or even gained some pounds.

## Q: Is this an easy diet to follow?

**A:** This depends upon the individual. The DASH diet does have some benefits that makes it easy to incorporate into your lifestyle. It happens to be very convenient as the recipe options are endless. There is always an option to eat healthy and keep it delicious at the same time. However, if you eat out often, it can make it a bit more difficult. If you find yourself at a restaurant, choose fruits and vegetables. Try your best to stay away from anything smoked, cured, or pickled.

## Q: How much exercise should I get?

**A:** The amount of exercise you do will depend on the individual. If you have no experience, we suggest starting out with about 15 minutes. Try to go for a walk around you block in the morning or at night. As you grow more comfortable, you can turn up the intensity and duration. You should never be uncomfortable with what you are doing. All you really need to do is find an activity you enjoy and then you can set your exercise goals around it!

## Q: Can I have sea salt instead of regular salt?

**A:** While sea salt may have slightly less sodium, it can still add up in your diet. Most times, the sea salt grains are smaller but have more weight per teaspoon. Instead, we suggest trying to season your foods with other herbs and spices. This way, you can keep as little salt in your diet as possible.

## Q: Should I be taking calcium, potassium, and magnesium supplements while on the DASH Diet?

**A:** This is not something we suggest. While many studies have been done on this subject, they found that taking these supplements will have no effect on lowering your blood pressure. It is best to just follow the diet and get the nutrients naturally!

## Q: Is there a vegetarian/ vegan version of the DASH Diet?

**A:** Luckily, most of the DASH diet is made of healthy vegan and vegetarian options. Beans, nuts, and seeds are all important parts of this diet. Any meat, fish, or poultry can have a non-animal alternative that is still rich in protein! If you are vegetarian or vegan, there are many recipes to keep the diet fun and delicious.

## Q: Can I still follow the diet if I am gluten intolerant?

**A:** Of course! If you have celiac disease or are gluten intolerant, you can still follow the DASH diet. All you will need to do is substitute any whole-wheat based foods for non-gluten options. Due to the fact that the diet contains mostly unprocessed foods, it makes it very easy to avoid any hidden gluten in products.

## Q: What spices can I use while on the DASH diet?

**A:** We are so glad you asked, here are some good ideas to spice up your diet!

Chicken - Sage, paprika, thyme, rosemary, ginger

Pork - Oregano, onion, garlic

Fish - curry powder, pepper, lemon juice, or dill

Vegetables - onion, pepper, parsley, sage, basil, marjoram

Sugar Substitute - cinnamon, unsweetened cocoa powder, dried fruits, applesauce

## Q: How can I stick with the DASH diet when eating out?

**A:** The DASH diet will work as long as you are determined. If you are out for a meal, try to choose a simple one where you can recognize the ingredients. You will also want to pay attention to serving sizes. Restaurants tend to give whopping portions. If possible, stick with any grilled or baked options. This way, you can usually avoid any foods that have a lot of fat.

## Q: Can I be on the DASH diet if I travel a lot?

**A:** Absolutely! All you have to do is pack the healthy food with you, or spend some extra time shopping on the road. This can be easily done with trail mixes and even fresh fruit. It may take some extra time, but at least you will always have it with you so you are never tempted by easy fast food!

## Q: How can I stick to the DASH diet in social situations?

**A:** If you are going to go out, try to schedule coffee dates instead of food dates. This way, you will not find yourself temped with high calorie foods. You can have a simple coffee either black or with skim milk. On nights out with friends or at events, try to eat beforehand so you're not tempted by any unhealthy snacks provided.

# Chapter 5:
# Breakfast Recipes

To help get you off to a smooth start with your DASH diet, here are some great breakfast recipes that you can try!

## Whole Wheat Pumpkin Pancakes (Serves 8)

Ingredients:

- 2 ½ Cups Whole-Wheat Pastry Flour
- 2 Tbsp. Baking Powder
- 2 Tsp. Ground Ginger
- 3 Tsp. Cinnamon
- ¼ Tsp. Ground Cloves
- ¼ Tsp. Nutmeg
- 2 Eggs
- 2 Cups Low-Fat Buttermilk
- 1 Cup Pumpkin Puree
- ¼ Cup Olive Oil

Instructions:

1. Combine flour, baking powder, ginger, nutmeg, cinnamon, cloves, and salt in a large bowl

2. Whisk together eggs, pumpkin puree, olive oil, and buttermilk in a separate bowl

3. Combine all ingredients together

4. Heat a pan on medium heat

5. Pour thin layer of mixture into the pan, and cook until bubble appear. Flip, and cook until golden on both sides

6. Serve

# Sweet Potato Cakes

Ingredients:

- 4 Cups Shredded & Peeled Sweet Potato
- ¼ Cup Whole Wheat Flour
- 1 Tsp. Instant Minced Onion
- 1/8 Tsp. Salt
- 1/8 Tsp. Pepper
- Dash of Ground Nutmeg
- 1 Large Egg, Slightly Beaten
- Cooking Spray

Instructions:

1. Combine all ingredients in a large bowl, and stir well
2. Coat a non-stick pan with cooking spray, and heat to medium-high
3. Spoon about ¼ cup of mixture onto the pan and flatten with a spatula. Cook for 4 minutes on each side or until golden brown
4. Serve

# Easy Omelet (Serves 4)

Ingredients:

- Cooking Spray
- 8 Eggs
- 2 Tbsp. Snipped Chives
- 1/8 Tsp. Salt
- 1/8 Tsp. Cayenne Pepper
- ½ Cup Reduced-Fat Cheddar Cheese
- 2 Cups Baby Spinach Leaves

Instructions:

1. Coat a 10-inch, nonstick pan with cooking spray and heat on medium.
2. Combine eggs, chives, salt, and pepper in a bowl.
3. Use a beater or whisk to mix the mixture until frothy
4. Pour into pan, and stir while it cooks until sections of cooked egg appear
5. Stop stirring and cook for an additional 30-60 seconds
6. Top with cheese and spinach
7. Fold one side of omelet over the filling
8. Serve

# Fruit Crunch (serves 6)

Ingredients:

- 4 Cups Assorted Fresh Fruit of Your Choice (peeled and diced)
- 12 Oz. of Low-Fat Vanilla Yogurt
- 2 Tbsp. Honey
- ½ Cup Low-Fat Granola Cereal
- ¼ Cup Toasted Coconut

Instructions:

1. Divide fruit among 6 tall parfait glasses, or bowls
2. Top fruit with yogurt, and drizzle with honey
3. Sprinkle with granola and coconut

## Stuffed Peaches (serves 8)

Ingredients:

- 4 Peaches, Halved & Pitted
- ½ Cup Dried Tropical Mixed Fruit
- ¼ Cup Slivered Almonds
- 2 Tbsp. Graham Cracker Crumbs
- 2 Tbsp. Brown Sugar
- ¼ Tsp. Ground Allspice
- 12 Oz. Peach Nectar
- ½ Cup Vanilla Yogurt

Instructions:

1. Preheat oven to 350F
2. Scoop out peach pulp to form a 2-inch circle in center of each half
3. Reserve pulp, and finely chop
4. Combine pulp, dried fruit, almonds, cracker crumbs, brown sugar, and allspice
5. Stuff peach halves with mixture
6. Place peach halves on a baking dish, and add nectar to the dish

7. Bake for 40 minutes or until peaches are tender

8. Drizzle peaches with nectar

## Easy Oatmeal (Serves 4)

Ingredients:

- 1 ½ Cups Fat-Free Milk
- 1 ½ Cups Water
- Cooking Spray
- 2 Gala Apples, Peeled & Cut into Small Cubes
- 1 Cup Uncooked, Steel-Cut Oats
- 2 Tbsp. Brown Sugar
- 1 ½ Tbsp. Softened Butter
- ¼ Tsp. Ground Cinnamon
- ¼ Tsp. Salt
- ¼ Cup Maple Syrup

Instructions:

1. Combine milk and water in a saucepan, and bring to a boil, stirring frequently
2. Coat a slow-cooker with cooking spray
3. Place hot mixture, plus all other ingredients (minus the maple syrup) into the slow cooker
4. Cover, and cook on low for 7 hours
5. Spoon oatmeal into bowls and top with maple syrup and hazelnuts (optional)

# Breakfast Melts (Serves 4)

Ingredients:

- 2 Whole Grain English Muffins, Split
- 1 Tsp. Olive Oil
- 8 Egg Whites, Whisked
- 4 Scallions, Finely Chopped
- Kosher Salt, to Taste
- Black Pepper, to Taste
- 2 Oz. Reduced-Fat Swiss Cheese, Shredded
- ½ Cup Cherry Heirloom Tomatoes, Quartered

Instructions:

1. Preheat the broiler on high
2. Place muffins, cut side up on a baking sheer, and broil for 2 minutes or until lightly brown on the edges
3. Heat a skillet on medium-heat
4. Add oil and sauté 3 of the scallions about 2-3 minutes
5. Add egg whites, season with salt & pepper, and mix until cooked through

6. Divide on toasted muffins, and top with tomatoes cheese, and remaining scallions

7. Broil for 1-2 minutes or until cheese has melted

8. Serve

# Avocado 'Toast' (Serves 1)

Ingredients:

- 2 Brown Rice Cakes
- ½ Avocado
- Small Tomato, Sliced
- Red Pepper Flakes
- Pinch of Salt

Instructions:

1. Mash avocado in a bowl with a fork
2. Spread evenly over rice cakes
3. Add tomato slices
4. Sprinkle with red pepper flakes and salt
5. Serve

## PB & J Yogurt (Serves 1)

Ingredients:

- 6 Oz. Fat-Free Plain Greek Yogurt
- 4 Tsp. Reduced Sugar Grape Jelly
- 2 Tsp. Red Seedless Grapes, Cut in Half
- 1 Tsp. Reduced-Fat Peanut Butter
- 1 Tsp. Unsalted Peanuts

Instructions:

1. Place the yogurt in a bowl
2. Top with jelly, then peanut butter
3. Lightly sprinkle peanuts and grape on top
4. Serve

## Quinoa Bowls (Serves 2)

Ingredients:

- 1 Small Peach, Sliced
- 1/3 Cup Uncooked Quinoa, Rinsed Well
- 2/3 Cup Low-Fat Milk
- ½ Tsp. Vanilla Extract
- 2 Tsp. Brown Sugar
- 12 Raspberries
- 14 Blueberries
- 2 Tsp. Honey

Instructions:

1. In a sauce pan, combine quinoa, 80% of the milk, vanilla, and brown sugar
2. Cook on medium heat, and bring to boil for 5 minutes
3. Reduce heat to low and cover for 15-20 minutes, or until it easily fluffs with a fork
4. Heat a grill pan and spray with oil
5. Grill the peaches for 2-3 minutes per side
6. Warm the remaining milk in the microwave

7. Divide the cooked quinoa between 2 bowls, then pour in warm milk

8. Top with peaches, raspberries, and blueberries

9. Drizzle with honey

10. Serve

# Chapter 6:
# Lunch & Dinner Recipes

## Vegetable Pasta Soup (Serves 12)

Ingredients:

- 2 Tsp. Olive Oil
- 6 Garlic Cloves (Minced)
- 1 ½ Cups Shredded Carrot
- 1 Cup Chopped Onion
- 1 Cup Thinly Sliced Celery
- 1 32-Ounce Box Reduced-Sodium Chicken Broth
- 4 Cups Water
- 1 ½ Cups Dried Pasta
- ¼ Cup Shaved Parmesan Cheese
- 2 Tbsp. Snipped Parsley

Instructions:

1. In a Dutch oven, heat oil over medium heat
2. Add garlic, and cook for 15 seconds
3. Add carrot, onion, and celery
4. Cook for 5-7 minutes or until tender, stirring occasionally

5. Add chicken broth to the water

6. Bring to the boil

7. Add uncooked pasta and cook for 7-8 minutes or until tender

8. Serve topped with parmesan cheese and parsley

# Skillet Sausage & Potatoes (Serves 6)

Ingredients:

- ½ Pound Cooked Smoked Turkey Sausage
- 3-4 Tbsp. Olive Oil
- 1 ¾ Lbs. Unpeeled, Red-Skinned Potatoes
- 2 Medium Onions
- 1 Tsp. Dried Thyme, Crushed
- 1 ½ Tsp. Cumin Seed
- ¼ Tsp. Salt
- ¼ Tsp. Pepper

Instructions:

1. Pour oil into heavy, ovenproof skillet and place directly on range top
2. Cut potatoes into small cubes, and cut onions into thin wedges
3. Cook potatoes and onion in skillet, uncovered, on medium heat for 12 minutes. Stir occasionally
4. Slice sausage into ¼ inch thick chunks
5. Add sausage to skillet. Add more oil if necessary to prevent sticking
6. Cook uncovered for 10 minutes, stirring often

7. Stir in thyme, cumin seed, salt, and pepper

8. Cook and stir for 1 minute additionally

9. Serve

# Chicken Salad Tacos (Serves 1)

Ingredients:

- 1/3 Cup Chopped/Shredded Cooked Chicken
- 2 Tbsp. Chopped Celery
- 1 Tbsp. Light Mayonnaise
- 1 Tbsp. Salsa
- 1 Tbsp. Shredded Cheddar Cheese
- 4 Mini Taco Shells

Instructions:

1. Combine chicken, celery, mayonnaise, salsa, and cheese in a bowl
2. Scoop mixture into taco shells
3. Serve

# Garlic-Rosemary Mushrooms (Serves 4)

Ingredients:

- 1 Oz. Bacon, Chopped
- 1 ½ Lbs. Mixed Mushrooms, Cut into ¼ Inch Slices
- 2 Medium Cloves, Finely Chopped
- 1 ½ Tsp. Chopped Rosemary
- ¼ Tsp. Salt
- Pepper, To Taste
- ¼ Cup Dry White Wine

Instructions:

1. Cook bacon in a large skillet over medium heat until it begins to brown
2. Add mushrooms, garlic, rosemary, salt, and pepper
3. Cook for 8-10 minutes or until almost dry, stirring occasionally
4. Pour in wine, and cook until most of the liquid has evaporated
5. Serve

# Chicken & Vegetable Salad (Serves 4)

Ingredients:

- ½ Cup Low-Fat Cottage Cheese
- 1 Tbsp. Catsup
- 1 Hard-Cooked Egg, Chopped
- 1 Tbsp. Thinly Slice Green Onion
- 1 Tbsp. Pickle Relish
- 1/8 Tsp. Salt
- 1 ½ Cups Cooked Chicken
- ½ Cup Chopped Celery
- ½ Cup Chopped Green Pepper
- Lettuce Leaves
- 2 Tsp. Toasted Sliced Almonds

Instructions:

1. Combine cottage cheese and catsup in a blender
2. Mix together cottage cheese mixture with egg, onion, pickle relish, and salt in a small bowl. Set aside
3. In a separate bowl, combine chicken, celery, and pepper
4. Combine both bowls and toss gently to mix

5. Cover and chill for 4 – 24 hours

6. Serve on a lettuce-lined plate

7. Garnish with almonds

# Spaghetti With Spinach (Serves 6)

Ingredients:

- 12 Oz. Spaghetti
- 4 Tbsp. Extra Virgin Olive Oil
- ½ Cup Bread Crumbs
- 4 Garlic Cloves, Minced
- ¼ Tsp. Red Pepper Flakes
- 6 Oz. Baby Spinach
- ½ Cup Grated Parmesan Cheese

Instructions:

1. Bring large pot of salted water to the boil, and cook spaghetti for about 12 minutes or until al dente
2. Heat 1 tbsp. of oil in a large non-stick skillet over medium-high heat
3. Add bread crumbs and cook for 2 minutes, stirring often
4. Add half of the garlic and half the red pepper flakes
5. Cook for 1 minute, stirring constantly. Remove from skillet and wipe clean
6. Reduce heat to low and add remaining 3 tbsp. oil, garlic, and red pepper flakes
7. Cook for 2 minutes or until garlic is golden

8. Add spinach to skillet and toss until wilted

9. Stir spinach mixture and parmesan cheese into pasta

10. Serve

# Marinated Fish Steaks (Serves 4)

Ingredients:

- 1 Lb. Fresh Salmon Steaks, Cut 1 Inch Thick
- 2 Tbsp. Lime Juice
- 1 Tbsp. Snipped Oregano
- 2 Tsp. Olive Oil
- 1 Tsp. Lemon-Pepper Seasoning
- 2 Cloves Garlic, Crushed
- 4 Lime Wedges

Instructions:

1. Rinse fish steaks and pat dry with paper towel
2. Cut into 4 serving size pieces (if necessary)
3. In a shallow dish, combine lime juice, oregano, lemon-pepper seasoning, and garlic
4. Add fish, and turn to coat
5. Cover and marinate in the fridge for 30 minutes – 2 hours
6. Drain fish, leaving the marinade
7. Place fish on the greased unheated rack of a broiler pan

8. Broil 4 inches from the heat for 8-12 minutes or until fish begins to flake when tested with a fork

9. Turn once and brush with leftover marinade halfway through cooking

10. Serve, and squeeze the juice of 1 lime wedge over each steak

# Raspberry Ginger Chicken (Serves 4)

Ingredients:

- 1 ¼ Lb. Chicken Breast Tenders
- 1 Tsp. Salt
- ¼ Tsp. Pepper
- 2 Tbsp. Olive Oil
- 1 Small Onion, Sliced
- 2 Cups Baby Carrots, Sliced
- 2 Cups Broccoli Florets
- 1 Tbsp. Seedless Raspberry Jam
- 1 Tbsp. White Wine Vinegar
- 1 Tbsp. Water
- 1 Tbsp. Soy Sauce
- 1 Tsp. Ground Ginger

Instructions:

1. Season chicken with salt and pepper
2. Heat oil over medium for 30 seconds in a large non-stick skillet
3. Add onion and carrots, and sauté for 5 minutes

4. Add broccoli and chicken, and sauté for 8 minutes more, turning occasionally until chicken is cooked

5. Remove chicken and vegetables to a large plate

6. In the same skillet, combine jam, vinegar, water, soy sauce and ginger

7. Whisk over low heat for 2 minutes

8. Add chicken and vegetables back in, and stir

9. Cook on low until chicken is very hot

10. Serve

# Chicken & Broccoli Stir Fry (Serves 4)

Ingredients:

- 1/3 Cup Orange Juice
- 1 Tbsp. Low-Sodium Soy Sauce
- 1 Tbsp. Schezuan Sauce
- 2 Tsp. Cornstarch
- 1 Tbsp. Canola Oil
- 1 Lb. Boneless Chicken (cut into 1 inch cubes)
- 2 Cups Frozen Broccoli Florets
- 6Oz Frozen Snow Peas
- 2 Cups Shredded Cabbage
- 2 Cups of Cooked Brown Rice
- 1 Tbsp. Sesame Seeds (optional)

Instructions:

1. Mix orange juice, soy sauce, schezuan sauce, and cornstarch in a small bowl. Set aside
2. Heat oil in wok and add chicken. Stir for 5-7 minutes or until done
3. Add cabbage, broccoli, snow peas, and sauce mixture. Cook for 5 minutes of until vegetables are heated through

4. Serve over brown rice with (optional) sesame seeds on top

## Turkey Loaf (Served 8)

Ingredients:

- 1 ½ Lbs. Lean Ground Turkey Breast
- 10 Oz. Frozen Chopped Spinach (thawed & drained)
- 1 Cup Quick Oats, Uncooked
- ½ Cup Finely Chopped Onions
- ½ Cup Shredded Carrots
- 2 Egg Whites
- 1/3 Cup Fat-Free Milk
- 1 ½ Tsp. Italian Seasoning Blend
- 1 Tsp. Salt
- ¼ Tsp. Black Pepper

Instructions:

1. Preheat oven to 350F
2. Combine all ingredients in a large bowl, mixing lightly
3. Form into a 9 x 5-inch loaf
4. Place loaf into a baking pan, or on rack of broiler pan

5. Bake for 1 hour

6. Let stand for 5 minutes, then serve

# Shepherd's Pie (Serves 6)

Ingredients:

- 2 Large Baking Potatoes, Peeled & Diced
- ½ Cup Low-Fat Milk
- 1 Pound Lean Ground Beef
- 1 Medium Onion, Chopped
- 1 Clove Garlic, Minced
- 2 Tbsp. Flour
- 4 Cups Frozen, Mixed Vegetables
- ¾ Cup Reduced Sodium Beef Broth
- ½ Cup Shredded Cheddar Cheese
- Ground Pepper to Taste

Instructions:

1. Put diced potatoes in a saucepan
2. Add enough water to barely cover. Bring to boil, then reduce heat and simmer, covered. Simmer until soft (about 15 minutes)
3. Drain potatoes and mash. Add milk, and set aside
4. Preheat oven to 375F
5. Brown meat, onion, and garlic in a large skillet

6. Stir in flour and cook for 1 minute, stirring constantly

7. Add vegetables and broth. Cook for 5 minutes or until bubbly, stirring well

8. Spoon vegetable mixture into square baking dish

9. Spread potato mixture over meat/vegetable mixture

10. Sprinkle cheese on top

11. Bake 25 minutes or until hot and bubbly

12. Serve

# Chapter 7:
# Smoothie Recipes

This chapter is dedicated to some great smoothie recipes that can be used as a breakfast replacement, for a snack, or just for when you're craving something sweet!

Simply blend all listed ingredients, and enjoy!

## Green Smoothie

Ingredients:

- 1 Medium Banana
- 1 Cup Baby Spinach
- ½ Cup Fat-Free Milk
- ¼ Cup Whole Oats
- ¾ Cup Frozen Mango
- ¼ Cup Plain Non-Fat Yogurt
- ½ Tsp. Vanilla

## Oatmeal Smoothie (Serves 2)

Ingredients:

- ½ Cup Ice
- 1 Banana
- 1 Cup Frozen Mixed Berries
- ½ Cup Plain, Low-Fat Yogurt
- ½ Cup Rolled Oats
- 1 Cup Low-Fat Milk
- 1 Tsp. Honey

# Chocolate Avocado Smoothie (Serves 2)

Ingredients:

- 2 Cups Vanilla Soy Milk
- ½ Avocado
- 1 Medium Banana
- ¼ Cup Unsweetened Cocoa Powder
- 2 Stevia Packets

# Almond Butter Smoothie

Ingredients:

- 7 Oz. Plain Greek Yogurt
- 1 Tbsp. Almond Butter
- ½ Banana
- ½ Tsp. Chia Seeds
- 1 Tbsp. Flaxseed Oil
- ½ Cup Ice

## Super Smoothie

Ingredients:

- ½ Cup Water
- ½ Cup Low Fat Yogurt
- ½ Cup Blueberries
- 1 Tbsp. Chia Seeds
- ½ Banana
- ½ Cup Ice

# Conclusion

Thanks again for taking the time to read this book!

You should now have a good understanding of the DASH Diet and be ready to try it out for yourself! Why not choose a few of the sample recipes, and dive right in!

If you enjoyed this book, please take the time to leave me a review on Amazon. I appreciate your honest feedback, and it really helps me to continue producing high quality books.

Made in the USA
Middletown, DE
04 January 2017